THE LOW-FODMAP FRUCTOSE INTOLERANCE COOKBOOK FOR BEGINNERS

Say Goodbye to Gastrointestinal Discomfort and Abdominal Pain, and Enjoy a Healthier Gut and Effective Weight Management

Chris Preston, RDN

ACKNOWLEDGEMENTS

I would like to express my deepest gratitude to everyone who supported me throughout the journey of creating this book. To my family and friends, your unwavering encouragement and patience have been invaluable.

A special thanks to my team, whose expertise and guidance were crucial in developing the dietary plans and recipes shared in this book. Your insights have been a cornerstone of this work.

I am also deeply grateful to my editor, Michael Jones, for your meticulous attention to detail and for helping shape this book into a comprehensive and accessible guide.

To the support groups and communities who shared their experiences and provided feedback, your contributions have enriched this book and made it more relatable for those living with fructose intolerance.

Lastly, to my readers, thank you for embarking on this journey with me. I hope this book provides you with the knowledge and tools to navigate your dietary needs and improve your quality of life.

COPYRIGHT

Copyright © Chris Preston, RDN. All rights reserved.

No part of this publication may be reproduced, distributed, or transmitted in any form or by any means, including photocopying, recording, or other electronic or mechanical methods, without the prior written permission of the publisher, except in the case of brief quotations embodied in critical reviews and certain other noncommercial uses permitted by copyright law.

This book is intended to provide general information about diet and nutrition. It is not intended as a substitute for professional medical advice, diagnosis, or treatment. Always seek the advice of your physician or other qualified health provider with any questions you may have regarding a medical condition.

Table of Contents

PART I

WHAT IS FRUCTOSE INTOLERANCE?

You thought you were making a smart, healthy choice with that fruit smoothie, but now your stomach feels like it's staging a protest. Could fructose intolerance be the culprit?

Fructose, a simple sugar naturally found in fruits, some vegetables, and honey, can turn from friend to foe for those with fructose intolerance. For these individuals, an innocent slice of watermelon or a handful of raisins can quickly become a day-wrecker.

Imagine enjoying a fresh fruit salad, only to be met with uncomfortable bloating, relentless gas, abdominal pain, and an urgent need for the bathroom. These are the hallmark symptoms of fructose intolerance. For those who can't properly digest fructose, such foods are a recipe for disaster.

There are two types of fructose intolerance: dietary fructose intolerance and the more severe hereditary fructose intolerance. While dietary fructose intolerance is challenging, hereditary fructose intolerance is a serious condition that manifests in infancy. If not managed correctly, it can lead to life-threatening complications like liver and kidney failure.

So, if your stomach is rebelling after that supposedly healthy snack, it might be time to consider if fructose intolerance is the hidden saboteur of your digestive peace.

Hereditary Fructose Intolerance: The Genetic Culprit

Imagine your body encountering a genetic glitch where the sweetest treats turn into a perilous trap. That's hereditary fructose intolerance (HFI), a genetic disorder where your body lacks a crucial enzyme called aldolase B, essential for breaking down fructose. This deficiency means your body struggles to digest fructose, found in various foods, leading to significant health challenges.

Causes

The root of hereditary fructose intolerance lies in your DNA. If both of your parents carry the faulty gene for aldolase B, you have a 25% chance of inheriting this condition. This enzyme, primarily located in the liver, is crucial for converting fructose into usable energy. Without it, your body can't metabolize fructose or sucrose (another type of sugar), causing your blood sugar to plummet and toxins to accumulate in your liver.

Symptoms

HFI often reveals itself in infancy, shortly after a baby starts consuming foods that contain fructose. Although new diagnoses in adults are rare, the symptoms are unmistakable and can be severe. Common signs include jaundice, stunted growth, vomiting, bloating, low phosphate and glucose levels in the blood, elevated fructose levels in the urine and blood, nausea, abdominal pain, and an aversion to fruit or sweet foods.

Complications

The consequences of undigested fructose building up in the body can be dire. HFI can lead to significant liver and kidney damage. In extreme cases, it can cause seizures, comas, and even organ failure. Other severe complications include gout, liver failure, internal bleeding, hypoglycemia (low blood sugar), and death.

For those living with hereditary fructose intolerance, careful management and dietary adjustments are crucial. Avoiding fructose-containing foods can help mitigate symptoms and prevent long-term damage, ensuring a better quality of life despite the challenges posed by this genetic disorder.

Dietary Fructose Intolerance: Understanding the Digestive Challenge

Dietary fructose intolerance, also known as fructose malabsorption, presents a common yet often misunderstood digestive issue. In this condition, the cells in your intestines struggle to absorb fructose properly, leading to a range of uncomfortable symptoms when fructose-rich foods are consumed.

Symptoms

Eating foods high in fructose can trigger symptoms similar to those of irritable bowel syndrome (IBS). These include:

Gas

Bloating

Diarrhea

Stomach pain

Causes and Development

Unlike hereditary fructose intolerance, which is genetic and presents from infancy, dietary fructose intolerance typically develops in adulthood. This condition arises when the intestine's ability to break down and absorb fructose becomes compromised. Various factors can exacerbate or contribute to this intolerance, such as celiac disease, Crohn's disease, gastroenteritis, inflammation, stress, and the use of antibiotics.

Management

Managing dietary fructose intolerance involves understanding your body's tolerance levels and making dietary adjustments accordingly. This may include reducing or avoiding foods high in fructose, such as certain fruits, sweeteners, and processed foods. Working with a healthcare professional, such as a dietitian, can help create a personalized plan to alleviate symptoms and improve digestive health.

Understanding the nuances of dietary fructose intolerance empowers individuals to make informed choices about their diet and lifestyle, ensuring better management of this common digestive challenge.

PART II

WHAT YOU SHOULD KNOW ABOUT FRUCTOSE?

Fructose is a type of sugar classified as a monosaccharide, meaning it exists as a single sugar molecule. It provides four calories per gram, similar to other sugars. Often referred to as "fruit sugar," fructose is naturally abundant in fruits, honey, sugar beets, sugar cane, and some vegetables. It holds the distinction of being the sweetest naturally occurring carbohydrate, 1.2–1.8 times sweeter than sucrose (table sugar). Unlike glucose, fructose metabolism does not rely on insulin and has minimal impact on blood glucose levels.

Origins and Forms

In nature, fructose commonly pairs with glucose to form sucrose, the typical table sugar. While fructose can exist as a standalone monosaccharide in plants, it never appears without other sugars. Its unique molecular structure contributes to its heightened sweetness compared to sucrose.

Health Considerations

Fructose can be a part of a balanced diet when consumed in its natural forms found in fruits, fruit juices, certain vegetables, and honey. However, concerns arise with its widespread inclusion in processed foods as high fructose corn syrup

(HFCS). HFCS, derived from corn starch, is added to sodas and candies, contributing to their sweetness but often lacking in nutritional value. These products should be consumed in moderation.

What We Know

The impact of excessive fructose consumption on human health remains contentious. While some studies suggest links between high fructose diets and conditions like obesity, diabetes, and certain cancers, moderation appears key. Current research aims to clarify these relationships and guide recommendations for optimal dietary practices.

Understanding the complexities of fructose allows individuals to make informed choices about their dietary intake, balancing enjoyment of its natural sweetness with considerations for overall health and wellness.

PART III

HOW FRUCTOSE WORKS IN OUR BODIES

Body cells require energy to carry out various processes, one of which is maintaining the "resting membrane potential." This potential allows cells to absorb substances from their surrounding fluid and facilitates cell-to-cell communication. Similar to glucose, fructose serves as an energy source for cells. Cells metabolize fructose to generate energy through aerobic respiration, a process that involves the oxidation of fructose in the presence of oxygen to produce ATP, the primary energy molecule for cellular activities.

Energy Storage and Utilization

Fructose isn't just used for immediate energy; it also plays a role in energy storage. The body converts fructose into glycogen, a storage carbohydrate composed of long chains of glucose. Glycogen is stored in the liver and muscles. The liver breaks down glycogen to release glucose into the bloodstream during periods of fasting or emergencies, ensuring a steady supply of glucose for all body cells. Muscle cells store glycogen for their own use, primarily during physical activity.

The partial breakdown of fructose yields compounds such as glyceraldehyde and dihydroxyacetone phosphate. These compounds are pivotal in glycogen synthesis. Glyceraldehyde can be converted into glyceraldehyde-3 phosphate, which, along with dihydroxyacetone phosphate, acts as a precursor in the formation of glycogen.

Fat Storage

Beyond glycogen, the body also stores energy in the form of triglycerides, commonly known as fat. Fat is a crucial energy reserve because it is both lightweight and energy-dense, allowing the body to store large amounts of energy without a significant increase in weight. Fructose can be chemically modified to produce precursors for fat synthesis, contributing to the body's ability to store energy efficiently.

Why Some People Can't Tolerate Fructose

When the digestive system fails to absorb fructose properly, it can lead to stomach pain, bloating, diarrhea, and gas — a condition known as fructose intolerance. People with fructose intolerance should limit their intake of high-fructose foods, including juices, apples, pears, watermelon, asparagus, and peas.

Fructose intolerance occurs when the body cannot properly digest and metabolize fructose. This can be due to a genetic mutation or develop for other reasons. While most people can convert fructose to glucose without issues, some individuals struggle with this process, making it difficult for their bodies to metabolize fructose effectively.

Most people can easily convert fructose to glucose without problems. However, for those who develop an intolerance, managing symptoms involves dietary adjustments and awareness of high-fructose foods to avoid.

Diagnosis, Managing and Treating Fructose Intolerance

For people with dietary fructose intolerance, there is no one-size-fits-all solution. "Most people can tolerate some fructose, but everyone has a different sensitivity to it," he says.

If you suspect fructose intolerance, your doctor will likely recommend an elimination diet. For several weeks, you won't consume any fructose. Then, you can slowly begin reintroducing fructose-containing foods to determine how much you can tolerate without experiencing symptoms.

Working with a dietitian during this process can be helpful to ensure you find what works for you and maintain adequate nutrition. Symptoms of fructose malabsorption typically occur when eating foods containing this sugar, indicating potential intolerance.

Doctors may perform a breath test to detect hydrogen levels in your breath, as high levels can suggest difficulty digesting fructose. An elimination diet can also diagnose malabsorption, where you avoid all foods containing fructose and other potential allergens and then monitor the results.

To diagnose hereditary fructose intolerance in babies, doctors can perform a liver biopsy to confirm a deficiency of aldolase or a feeding test where fructose is delivered through an IV needle, and the body's response is assessed. These methods may be risky, so a DNA test is a safer alternative that can suggest fructose intolerance without the dangers of traditional testing.

For people with hereditary fructose intolerance, it's recommended to avoid consuming any fructose-containing foods. One case study reported a woman developing symptoms after just one sip of a sweetened beverage. People with dietary fructose intolerance should follow a low-fructose diet, avoiding high-fructose foods and incorporating those low in fructose. The exact amount of fructose that can be consumed without symptoms will vary among individuals.

Generally, the symptoms of fructose intolerance can be well managed through careful eating habits.

PART IV

CHANGING YOUR DIET

Foods to Avoid

If you have fructose intolerance, it's essential to avoid foods and drinks high in fructose. Fructose is commonly found in fruits and in high-fructose corn syrup, a sweetener used in many products. Here are some guidelines and examples of foods to avoid and alternatives you can enjoy.

Foods to Avoid

Sweeteners:

Agave nectar

Honey

High-fructose corn syrup

Maple syrup

Molasses

Palm sugar

Coconut sugar

Beverages:

Fruit juices

Sodas

Sweetened drinks

Fruits:

Apples

Grapes

Watermelon

Mangoes

Tomatoes

Dried fruits (e.g., prunes, raisins, dates)

Fruits canned in juice or syrup

Fruit purees like applesauce

Fruit jams or jellies

Vegetables:

Artichokes

Asparagus

Broccoli

Leeks

Mushrooms

Okra

Onions

Peas

Red peppers

Shallots

Zucchini

Other Foods:

Foods with wheat as the main ingredient (e.g., wheat bread, pasta)

Meats marinated or seasoned with fructose-containing ingredients

Desserts sweetened with fructose

High-fructose corn syrup is a common sweetener in many processed foods, from yogurt to soda. Always read labels carefully to identify hidden sources of fructose.

Lower-Fructose Alternatives

Fortunately, there are fruits and foods with lower fructose content that some people with dietary fructose intolerance can tolerate better. These include:

Avocados

Bananas

Cranberries

Cantaloupe

Lemons and limes

Oranges

Pineapple

Strawberries

Managing fructose intolerance involves careful selection and moderation of foods. By avoiding high-fructose foods and opting for lower-fructose alternatives, you can minimize symptoms and maintain a balanced diet.

Safe Foods to Eat

For those with dietary fructose intolerance, incorporating fruits and vegetables low in fructose can help manage symptoms while still enjoying a nutritious diet. Here are some options that are generally better tolerated:

Fruits:

Bananas

Cranberries

Kiwi

Lime

Mandarin oranges

Pineapple

Strawberries

Vegetables:

Carrots

Celery

Chives

Green peppers

White potatoes

Winter squash

Additional Low-Fructose Choices:

Citrus fruits like lemons, limes, and oranges

Avocados

Berries such as blueberries and cranberries

Lettuce

Green beans

Cantaloupe

Try to incorporate these low-fructose fruits and
vegetables into your diet to maintain a balanced

and varied nutritional intake. These foods can be included in salads, smoothies, snacks, and as side dishes to your meals. By focusing on low-fructose options, you can enjoy a diverse range of flavors and nutrients without triggering uncomfortable symptoms.

PART V

DELICIOUSLY SIMPLE LOW-FODMAP RECIPES YOU MUST TRY!

LOW-FODMAP RECIPES FOR BREAKFAST

Low FODMAP Chilli Oil and Feta Eggs

Cook Time: 2-5 minutes

Serves: 1

Ingredients:

2 eggs

1 tbsp cooking olive oil

¼ tsp chilli flakes

1 tbsp crumbled feta cheese

1 tbsp chopped green onions (optional)

Salt and ground pepper to taste

Gluten free or sourdough bread (optional) (e.g. Alpine bread)

Preparations

1. Heat olive oil in a pan over medium heat. Once the oil is hot, add chilli flakes and swirl for a few seconds to release the flavor. Optionally, stir in spring onions.

2. Crack the eggs into the pan and fry them according to your preference.

3. If you prefer your eggs flipped, do so now. Then, crumble feta cheese on top of the eggs. Serve immediately.

4. Optionally, toast 1-2 slices of bread in the same pan using the residual oil for extra flavor.

5. Serve the eggs on top of your toast and enjoy!

Low FODMAP Hot Cross Buns

Prep time: 2 hrs (including rising time)

Cook Time: 15-20 minutes

Serves: 12

<u>Ingredients:</u>

For the Buns:

– 2 cups gluten-free all-purpose flour

– 1/2 cup almond flour

– 1/4 cup unsalted butter, melted

- 1/2 cup lactose-free milk (or almond milk)

- 1/4 cup pure maple syrup

- 2 large eggs

- 1 packet (2 1/4 tsp) active dry yeast

- 1 tsp ground cinnamon

- 1/2 tsp ground nutmeg

- 1/2 tsp salt

- Zest of one orange

For the Cross:

- 1/4 cup gluten-free all-purpose flour

- 3-4 tbsp water

For the Glaze:

- 2 tbsp pure maple syrup

<u>Preparations</u>

1. In a small bowl, combine the yeast with a tablespoon of maple syrup and warm lactose-free milk. Let it sit for 5-10 minutes until frothy.

2. In a large mixing bowl, combine the gluten-free all-purpose flour, almond flour, melted butter, remaining maple syrup, eggs, cinnamon, nutmeg, salt, and orange zest. Add the activated yeast mixture.

3. Knead the dough on a floured surface until smooth. Place it in a greased bowl, cover with a damp cloth, and let it rise in a warm place for 1-2 hours or until doubled in size.

4. Preheat the oven to 375°F (190°C). Line a baking tray with parchment paper.

5. Divide the dough into 12 equal portions and shape them into buns. Place them on the prepared tray.

6. Mix the gluten-free all-purpose flour with water to create a thick paste. Pipe a cross onto each bun.

7. Bake in the preheated oven for 15-20 minutes or until the buns are golden brown.

8. While the buns are still warm, brush them with pure maple syrup for a glossy finish.

9. Allow the buns to cool slightly before serving. Enjoy your Low FODMAP Hot Cross Buns!

Low FODMAP Turkey Lettuce Wraps

Prep time: 20 minutes

Cook time: 15 minutes

Serves: 4

<u>Ingredients:</u>

- 500 grams cooked leftover turkey

- 1 tablespoon low FODMAP soy sauce or tamari (e.g. San J sauce range)

- 1 tablespoon rice vinegar

- 1 teaspoon grated ginger

- 1/2 teaspoon red pepper flakes (optional)

- 1 head of lettuce (such as iceberg or butter lettuce), leaves separated

- 1 cucumber, thinly sliced

- 1 carrot, grated

- Fresh cilantro leaves, for garnish (optional)

- Lime wedges, for serving

For the Dipping Sauce:

- 2 tablespoons low FODMAP soy sauce or tamari

- 1 tablespoon maple syrup

– 1 tablespoon rice vinegar

– 1 teaspoon sesame oil (optional)

– 1/2 teaspoon grated ginger

Preparations

1. In a small bowl, whisk together the low FODMAP soy sauce (or tamari), rice vinegar, grated ginger, and red pepper flakes (if using). Set aside

2. Heat the turkey in a large pan or skillet over medium-low heat.

3. Pour the sauce over the cooked turkey and stir to coat evenly. Heat for an additional 2-3 minutes to allow the flavours to meld together.

4. Meanwhile, prepare the dipping sauce by whisking together the low-FODMAP soy sauce (or tamari), maple syrup, rice vinegar, sesame oil (if using), and grated ginger in a small bowl.

5. To assemble the lettuce wraps, take a lettuce leaf and spoon some of the cooked turkey onto it. Top with cucumber slices, grated carrot, and cilantro leaves (if desired). Drizzle with the dipping sauce and squeeze a fresh lime wedge over the filling.

6. Repeat with the remaining lettuce leaves and filling ingredients.

7. Serve the turkey lettuce wraps as a refreshing and flavorful low FODMAP meal.

Enjoy!

Low FODMAP Pumpkin Spice Latte

Prep time: 5 minutes

Cook time: 5 minutes

Serves: 2

<u>Ingredients:</u>

2 cups lactose-free milk (or low FODMAP milk of choice)

2 tablespoons canned pumpkin puree (ensure no added sugars)

2 tablespoons pure maple syrup

1/2 teaspoon pumpkin pie spice blend (combine ground ginger, nutmeg and cinnamon)

1/2 teaspoon pure vanilla extract

1 cup strong brewed coffee (or espresso)

Whipped lactose-free cream (optional, for topping)

Ground cinnamon (optional, for garnish)

<u>Preparations</u>

1. In a small saucepan, combine the lactose-free milk, canned pumpkin puree, and pure maple syrup over medium-low heat. Whisk together until well combined.

2. Add the pumpkin pie spice blend and pure vanilla extract to the milk mixture. Continue to heat, stirring occasionally, until the mixture is steaming but not boiling.

3. While the milk mixture is heating, brew a cup of strong coffee or espresso.

4. Once the milk mixture is heated through, remove it from the heat and use a hand blender or a regular blender to blend it until frothy.

5. Divide the brewed coffee or espresso between two mugs.

6. Pour the frothy pumpkin spice milk mixture over the coffee in each mug.

7. Enjoy!

Optional: Top with whipped lactose-free cream and a sprinkle of ground cinnamon for extra indulgence.

NOTE: Although, coffee is not a FODMAP, caffeine can be a common gut irritant. As we are all different and have different tolerances, it is good to assess your own tolerance.

Low FODMAP Greek Salad Wrap

Prep time: 15 minutes

Serves: 2

Ingredients:

– 2 gluten-free wraps or large lettuce leaves

- 1/2 cucumber, diced

- 1/2 cup cherry tomatoes, halved

- 15 olives, pitted and sliced

- 40g crumbled feta cheese (omit for a dairy-free or vegan option)

- 2 tablespoons extra-virgin olive oil

- 1 tablespoon red wine vinegar

- 1 teaspoon dried oregano

- Salt and pepper, to taste

- Beef, Chicken or Lamb (omit for a dairy-free or vegan option)

Preparations

1. In a medium bowl, combine the cucumber, cherry tomatoes, olives, feta cheese (if desired), extra-virgin olive oil, red wine vinegar, dried oregano, salt, and pepper. Toss well to combine.2.

Lay out the gluten-free wraps or lettuce leaves on a clean surface.3. Spoon the Greek salad mixture onto the centre of each wrap or lettuce leaf, top with your meat of choice (if desired).

4. Fold in the sides of the wrap or lettuce leaf, then roll it up tightly, similar to a burrito, ensuring the filling is secure.

5. Slice the wrap in half if desired, and serve immediately.

6. Enjoy the vibrant flavours and crisp textures of the Greek Salad Wrap. It's a refreshing and satisfying option that brings together the classic elements of a Greek salad in a convenient handheld form.

Low FODMAP Choc Peanut Energy Balls

Prep time: 15 mins

Serves: 12 Energy Balls

<u>Ingredients:</u>

1 cup gluten-free rolled oats

1/2 cup smooth peanut butter (look for a brand without added high FODMAP ingredients)

1/4 cup maple syrup

2 tbsp unsweetened cocoa powder

1/4 cup dark chocolate chips (make sure they are low FODMAP)

1/4 cup unsweetened shredded coconut (optional, for rolling)

<u>Preparations</u>

1. In a large mixing bowl, combine the oats, peanut butter, maple syrup, cocoa powder, and dark chocolate chips. Stir until well combined.

2. Using clean hands, roll the mixture into small balls, about 1 inch in diameter.

3. If desired, roll the energy balls in shredded coconut to coat.

4. Place the energy balls in an airtight container and refrigerate for at least 30 minutes to firm up.

5. Serve chilled and enjoy as a delicious low-FODMAP dessert or a snack on-the-go!

Low FODMAP Smashed Pumpkin on Sourdough Toast

Prep time: 20 mins

Cook time: 40 mins

Serves: 1

Ingredients:

90g Butternut Pumpkin

1/4 cup or 40g canned chickpeas

1 tsp paprika

2 slices of Sourdough bread of your choice

5 tsp Extra-virgin olive oil

1 tsp Lemon juice to season

Salt and pepper to season

Preparations

1. Preheat oven to 180ºC

2. Thinly slice pumpkin and place in microwave friendly bowl. Cover with lid and microwave for 8 minutes on medium.

3. Prepare chickpeas by combining chickpeas with nutmeg, 1 tsp olive oil and a pinch of salt in a bowl. Spread onto a third of the oven tray.

4. Remove steamed pumpkin from the microwave friendly bowl and onto remaining space on the oven tray. Drizzle pumpkin with 2 tsp olive oil and place the tray in the oven.

5. Roast in the oven for 20 minutes, or until chickpeas and pumpkin form a golden-brown crust.

6. Toast sourdough bread in the oven grill or in a toaster until golden. Lightly drizzle with remaining olive oil. Layer roast pumpkin onto

toast and smash with the back of a fork. Top with roast chickpeas and sprinkle with fresh lemon juice. Serve.

7. Option to add fried halloumi and basil as a complimentary side.

Low FODMAP Bruschetta

Prep time: 10 mins

Cook time: 5 mins

Serves: 1

Ingredients:

2 slices of sourdough bread

250g cherry tomatoes

½ tsp Garlic infused extra virgin olive oil

½ tsp Extra virgin olive oil

¼ bunch Fresh basil

1 tsp White wine vinegar

Salt and pepper

<u>Preparations</u>

1. Slice the cherry tomatoes into halves or quarters and place in a bowl.

2. Lightly drizzle with garlic infused olive oil, white wine vinegar and season with salt and pepper to taste.

3. Tear in basil leaves and toss.

4. Toast bread on barbeque or griddle pan until lightly charred.

5. Lightly drizzle olive oil over the top of the toast and heap with the cherry tomato mixture. Option to lightly scrunch tomatoes with hands before placing on the toast.

6. Option to serve with your choice of cheese.

Low FODMAP Chocolate Chia Pudding

Prep Time: 5 minutes

Chill time: 2 hours

Serves: 4

Ingredients:

1 cup unsweetened almond milk

7 TBS chia seeds

3 TBS unsweetened cocoa powder

2 TBS maple syrup

1 TSP vanilla extract

Low-FODMAP toppings of your choice, such as berries, nuts, or dark chocolate chips

Preparations

1. In a medium bowl, whisk together the almond milk, chia seeds, cocoa powder, maple syrup, and vanilla extract.

2. Divide the mixture evenly among four jars or cups.

3. Cover the jars or cups and refrigerate for at least 2 hours, or until the pudding has thickened.

4. When ready to serve, top each pudding with your favourite low-FODMAP toppings

Low FODMAP One-Pot Tomato and Chicken Pasta

Prep time: 10 mins

Cook time: 20 mins

Serves: 4

<u>Ingredients:</u>

1 pound boneless, skinless chicken breast, cut into bite-sized pieces

2 tbsp olive oil

1 tsp FreeFOD Onion Replacer

2 tsp FreeFOD Garlic Replacer

2 cups cherry tomatoes, halved

1 cup chicken broth

1 cup gluten-free pasta

Salt and pepper, to taste

Fresh basil leaves, for garnish

<u>Preparations</u>

1. In a large skillet, heat the olive oil over medium heat. Add the chicken and cook until golden brown, about 5-7 minutes.

2. Add the onion and garlic replacers to the skillet and cook for another minute.

3. Add the cherry tomatoes, chicken broth, gluten-free pasta, salt, and pepper to the skillet. Stir to combine and bring the mixture to a boil.

Reduce heat to low, cover the skillet, and let the pasta cook for 10-12 minutes, or until the pasta is tender and the liquid has been absorbed.

Serve the pasta hot, garnished with fresh basil leaves if desired.

Low FODMAP Banana Oat Pancakes

Prep time: 5 mins

Cook time: 10 mins

Serves: 1

Ingredients:

1 Firm/unripe banana

1 tsp Baking power

1/3 cup Rolled oats

1/3 cup Lo-Fo plain flour (or other low FODMAP flour)

1 Egg

1 tsp Olive oil

Preparations

1. Mash banana into a bowl.

2. Sift baking powder and Lo-Fo plain flour into a bowl, then mix with rolled oats and egg.

3. Grease a non-stick pan with olive oil and heat on the stove.

4. Use ¼ cup mixture per pancake and dollop on the stove. Cook until small bubbles form on the top of the pancakes. Flip and then continue cooking until the underside is golden brown. Grease the pan in between batches of pancakes.

5. Serve with maple syrup or low FODMAP jam.

Low FODMAP Yoghurt Parfait

Prep Time: 5 minutes

Serves: 1

Ingredients:

3/4 cups Lactose-free Yoghurt (e.g. Jalna Strawberry Yoghurt or Liddells Tropical Yoghurt)

½ cup chopped low FODMAP fruits (berries, unripe banana, green kiwi)

¼ cup low FODMAP granola (e.g. Fodilicious Double Choco Granola)

Drizzle of maple syrup (optional)

Preparations

1. Add a layer of yoghurt to the bottom of a glass jar or bowl.

2. Then, add a layer of the low FODMAP granola followed by fruit

3. Repeat until the ingredients are used up.

4. Drizzle with maple syrup if desired.

5. Serve immediately to enjoy the crunchy granola.

Low FODMAP Berry Smoothie

Prep time: 10 mins

Serves: 2

Ingredients:

– 1 cup mixed berries (such as strawberries and blueberries)

– 1 unripe banana

– 1 cup lactose-free yoghurt

– 1 tablespoon chia seeds

– 1 tablespoon pure maple syrup

– 1 cup ice cubes

Preparations

1. In a blender, combine the mixed berries, ripe banana, lactose-free yoghurt, chia seeds, and pure maple syrup.

2. Add the ice cubes to the blender.

3. Blend on high speed until the ingredients are well combined and the smoothie reaches your desired consistency.

4. Taste the smoothie and adjust the sweetness by adding more maple syrup if needed.

5. Pour the smoothie into a glass.

6. Optional: Garnish with a few extra berries on top for an extra burst of freshness.

7. Serve immediately and enjoy your Low FODMAP Berry Smoothie!

LOW-FODMAP RECIPES FOR LUNCH

Low FODMAP Quinoa Stuffed Peppers

Prep time: 15 mins

Cppk time: 25 mins

Serves: 2

Ingredients:

- 2 green bell peppers, halved and cleaned

- 1 cup cooked quinoa

- 250g (1/2 lb) ground turkey or lean ground beef

- 1/2 cup diced tomatoes

- 2 green onions (green parts only), chopped

- Feta cheese, crumbled (optional)

– Fresh herbs (parsley or basil)

– Salt and pepper

<u>Preparations</u>

1. Preheat the oven to 190°C (375°F).

2. In a skillet, cook the ground turkey or beef until browned. Drain excess fat.

3. In a large bowl, mix cooked quinoa, browned meat, diced tomatoes, green onions, and salt and pepper.

4. Stuff each pepper half with the quinoa mixture.

5. Top with crumbled feta cheese if desired.

6. Bake in the preheated oven for 25 minutes or until peppers are tender.

7. Garnish with fresh herbs before serving.

8. Enjoy your Low FODMAP Quinoa Stuffed Peppers!

Low FODMAP Chicken Fajitas (GF)

Prep Time: 25 minutes

Cook Time: 20 minutes

Serves: 6

Ingredients:

3 Boneless chicken breasts

3 Red Capsicums

150g Broccoli heads

¼ tsp Chili powder

½ tsp Cumin

1 tsp Smoked paprika

1 tsp oregano

1 tbsp Spring onion, diced (Green parts only)

1 Lime

1 tbsp Extra-virgin olive oil

Salt and Pepper

For Serving

Gluten Free Tortillas

1 Tomato, diced

1 Avocado, diced

Lactose Free Sour Cream

Preparations

1. Create the fajita seasoning by combining Chili powder, cumin, smoked paprika, and oregano into a small bowl.

2. Finely slice chicken breasts into 2 x 8 cm pieces. Generously cover chicken with fajita seasoning, using your fingers.

3. Dice capsicums and broccoli heads.

4. Brown chicken on high with a frying pan, then turn down to medium for 10-15 minutes or until chicken is cooked through and golden in colour.

5. Remove chicken from the pan and fry vegetables in the same pan on medium heat, collecting as much of the flavour/seasoning from the sides of the pan as possible. When Vegetables are charred and golden brown, remove the pan from the heat and add chicken and lime juice. Lightly toss Chicken and vegetables before serving.

6. Option to serve with lactose free cream cheese, fresh tomato and avocado on a gluten free tortilla to serve.

Low FODMAP Veggie Frittata Recipe (GF)

Prep Time: 10 minutes

Cook time: 25 minutes

Serves: 4

<u>Ingredients:</u>

1 tbsp olive oil

1 cup diced low-FODMAP vegetables (Such as spinach, capsicum, tomato etc – Throw in anything you like, it's a great way to use up the leftover veg in the frigde!)

8 large eggs

1/4 cup unsweetened almond milk

Salt and pepper, to taste

1/4 cup grated cheese (either cheddar or mozzarella)

Fresh herbs (optional, for garnish)

Preparations

1. Preheat your oven to 400°F (200°C).

2. In an oven-safe skillet, heat the olive oil over medium heat. Add the diced low-FODMAP vegetables and cook until tender, about 5-7 minutes.

3. In a large bowl, whisk together the eggs, almond milk, salt, and pepper.

4. Pour the egg mixture over the cooked vegetables in the skillet. Sprinkle the grated cheese over the top.

5. Transfer the skillet to the oven and bake for 15-20 minutes, or until the frittata is set and the cheese is melted.

6. Remove the frittata from the oven and let it cool for a few minutes. Slice into four portions and serve warm, garnished with fresh herbs if desired.

Low FODMAP Quinoa and Vegetable Bowl (GF)

Prep Time: 10 minutes

Prep Time: 20 minutes

Serves: 4

Ingredients:

1 cup quinoa

2 cups water

1 tbsp olive oil

1 cup diced low-FODMAP vegetables of choice (such as carrots, green capsicum, broccoli, sweet potato etc.)

Salt and pepper, to taste

1/4 cup sliced low-FODMAP nuts (such as walnuts, peanuts)

2 tbsp freshly squeezed lemon juice

Fresh herbs (optional, for garnish)

<u>Preparations</u>

1. Rinse the quinoa thoroughly and place it in a medium saucepan along with 2 cups of water. Bring the water to a boil, then reduce the heat to low and let the quinoa cook, covered, for 18-20 minutes or until the water has been absorbed.

2. While the quinoa is cooking, heat the olive oil in a large skillet over medium heat. Add the diced vegetables and cook until tender, about 5-7 minutes. Season with salt and pepper to taste.

3. When the quinoa is finished cooking, fluff it with a fork and divide it evenly among four bowls.

4. Top each bowl with the cooked vegetables and sliced low-FODMAP nuts.

4. Drizzle each bowl with lemon juice and garnish with fresh herbs if desired and enjoy!

Low FODMAP Pad Thai Noodles

Prep Time: 15 minutes

Cook time: 15 minutes

Serves: 4

<u>Ingredients:</u>

300g packet of Mrs. Tran's Kitchen Flat Rice Noodles

1 Large Chicken Breast – Sliced (200g)

200g Firm Tofu

200g Raw Prawn Cutlets

2 Eggs – Whisked

1 Cup Bean Sprouts

½ Cup Chives or Spring Onions (green parts only) – cut 5cm pieces

Garlic Infused Oil or Vegetable Oil

Pad Thai Sauce:

2 Tsp Tamarind Paste (substitute with Rice Wine Vinegar if unavailable)

1 Tbsp Gluten Free Soy Sauce

2 Tbsp Gluten Free Fish Sauce

2 Tbsp Brown Sugar

Optional Garnishes:

Lime Wedges

Crushed Peanuts

Coriander Sprigs

Dried Chilli Flakes

Preparations

1. Cook the Flat Rice Noodles as per packet instructions.

2. Mix Pad Thai Sauce ingredients together and set aside.

3. On high heat in a wok or large frypan, add 1 tbsp of oil as desired. Add chicken, cook for about 2 minutes then add prawns and tofu. Cook for

another 2 minutes or until chicken & prawns are just cooked through. Remove from wok/pan and keep aside.

4. Add whisked eggs to wok and cook for 1 minute, breaking cooked eggs into large chunks and remove from wok once cooked.

5. Turn heat down to medium and add 1 tbsp oil to coat wok. Add noodles and prepared sauce and mix well.

6. Add back chicken, prawns, tofu and eggs and mix thoroughly. Turn off the heat, add bean sprouts, garlic chives/spring onions, squeeze a wedge of lime over noodles and lightly toss to mix.

7. Serve immediately with some extra bean sprouts, garlic chives, coriander and a wedge of lime.

Optional: crushed peanuts and dried chilli flakes.

Low FODMAP Slow Cooked Lamb Shanks

Prep Time: 10 minutes

Cook time: 5-9 hours hours

Serves: 4

Ingredients:

- 4 lamb shanks– 2 tbsp olive oil– 1 tsp FreeFOD Onion Replacer

- 2 tbsp tomato purée

- 250ml light red wine (such as pinot noir)

- 2 tbsp LoFo Pantry Low FODMAP plain flour

- 2 tsp San Elk Vegetable stock mixed into 500ml hot water

– 2 carrots, chopped

– 1 tsp FreeFOD Garlic Replacer

– 2 bay leaves

– 2 thyme sprigs

– 1 bunch parsley, leaves chopped separately to the stalks

Preparations

1. If needed, pre-heat your slow cooker.

2. In a large hot frying pan, add half the oil and brown the lamb shanks all over, then transfer them to the slow cooker.

3. This will take you about 10 mins and you may need to do it in batches.

3. Add the remaining oil to the frying pan and the onion replacer, then stir in the tomato purée and flour and cook for a minute.

4. Add the red wine and bring it to a boil, stirring the flour and purée into the wine until you have a smooth sauce.

5. Tip into the slow cooker. Pour the stock into the same pan and bring it to a boil, then tip into the slow cooker.

6. Add the carrots, garlic replacer, bay leaves, thyme and parsley stalks to the slow cooker and put the lid on.

7. Cook on low for eight hours or on high for four hours. Turn the shanks over at some point during the cooking.

8. After eight hours the lamb should be tender and starting to fall off the bone.

Note: If the sauce is too thin lift out the lamb and carrots and tip the sauce into a pan, boil it rapidly until it starts to thicken before adding the parsley.

9. Serve and enjoy!

Low FODMAP Quesadilla – Chicken, Beef or Vegetarian

Prep Time: 10 minutes

Cook time: 15 minutes

Serves: 2

<u>Ingredients:</u>

QUESADILLAS:

- 4 x La Tortilleria Corn Tortilla's

- 100g Liddells lactose free pizza cheese blend or Green Valley Creamery Lactose Free Shredded Mozzarella

– 1/4 cup roughly chopped coriander/cilantro

– 100g fresh sweet corn kernels (skin removed and cut from cob)

QUESADILLA SPICE MIX:

– 1/2 tsp dried oregano

– 1/2 tsp salt

– 1 tsp cumin powder

– 1 tsp paprika

– Pinch of black pepper, cayenne pepper (optional if you like spicy)

QUESADILLA FILLING:

– 1 tsp olive oil

– 1 tsp FreeFOD low FODMAP garlic replacer

– 1 tsp FreeFOD low FODMAP onion replacer

– 50g red capsicum/bell peppers, diced

– 1 tbsp tomato paste

Choose one filling of choice:

– 200g beef mince or,

– 200g chicken breast/tenderloin or,

– 1/4 can of black beans, drained

Preparations

1. In a small bowl, mix together all ingredients for the spice mix.

2. Cook your chosen quesadilla filling:

Beef filling

1. Heat oil in a skillet over high heat. Add onion and garlic replacer, cook for 2 minutes.

2. Add beef and cook, breaking it up as you go. Once it changes from pink to brown, add capsicum. Cook for 1 minute.

3. Add tomato paste, water and spice mix. Cook for 2 minutes.

4. Transfer to bowl, cool.

Chicken filling

1. Cut up chicken into small pieces.

2. Drizzle chicken with 1 tbsp oil, toss to coat. sprinkle over spice mix, toss well to coat.

3. Heat 1 tbsp oil in a large skillet over medium heat. Add chicken and cook for 3 minutes until deep golden.

4. Add onion and garlic replacer. Turn and cook chicken for 3 minutes until cooked through.

4. Add capsicum and cook for 1 minute.

5. Transfer to bowl, cool.

Vegetable filling

i.   Heat oil in a skillet over high heat.

ii.   Add capsicum and the onion and garlic replacer, cook for 1 minute.

iii.   Add beans, tomato paste, water and spice mix. Cook for 2 minutes.

iv.   Transfer to bowl, cool.

3. Preheat non stick skillet over medium low heat (if pan is not non-stick use 2 tsp oil).

4. Place tortilla on work surface. Sprinkle one side with a bit of cheese, top with filling of choice.

5. Sprinkle with corn, coriander and top with cheese, then, fold in half.

6.. Place quesadilla in skillet, press down lightly, cover with lid. Cook for 3 minutes until underside is super golden brown and crispy.

7. Carefully flip over the folded edge. Press down lightly. Cook for 3 minutes until crispy (no lid).

8. Transfer to cutting board, cut in half. Serve immediately!

Low FODMAP Smoked Salmon Poke Bowl

Prep Time: 5 minutes

Cook time: 10 minutes

Serves: 2

Ingredients:

– 100g smoked salmon

– 100g edamame beans

– Beetroot, shaved

– 50g Fresh corn off the cob and toasted

– ¼ avocado, sliced

– ¼ cup coriander, chopped

– 100g rice, cooked

– 1 tbsp sesame seeds, toasted

– 2 tbsp San-J Gluten Free Tamari Soy Sauce

– 1 tsp rice vinegar

– 1 tsp sesame oil

– 1 tsp fresh ginger, grated

Preparations

1. To make dressing, combine soy sauce, rice vinegar, sesame oil and ginger.

2. Arrange the rice at the bottom of the bowl.

3. Arrange all other ingredients on top and serve with dressing mixed through.

4. Garnish with coriander and sesame seeds and enjoy!

Low FODMAP Christmas Maple Glazed Ham

Prep Time: 30 minutes

Cook time: 2 hours

Serves: 30 people

<u>Ingredients:</u>

5 kg / 10 lb leg ham, bone in, skin on

30 Cloves (for studding the ham, optional – mainly for decorative purposes)

2 oranges , cut into quarters (Note 2)

 cup (250ml) water

GLAZE

3/4 cup (185ml) maple syrup

3/4 cup (165g) brown sugar , packed

3 tbsp dijon mustard

3/4 tsp ground cinnamon

1/2 tsp All Spice

<u>Preparations</u>

Resting time 20 minutes

1. Take ham out of fridge 1 hour prior.

2. Preheat oven to 160°C / 320°F (140°C fan). Arrange shelf in lower third so the ham will be sitting in the centre of the oven (rather than in top half of oven).

3. Place the Glaze ingredients in a bowl and mix until combined – use whisk if needed.

REMOVE HAM RIND (SKIN)

4. Run small knife around bone handle, down each side of the ham, and under the rind on the cut face. (See video & photos in post)

5. Slide fingers under the rind on the cut face of the ham, and run them back and forth to loosen while pulling the rind back. Use knife if needed to slice off any residual rind.

6. Lightly cut 2.5cm / 1" diamonds across the fat surface of the ham, about 75% of the way into the fat. Avoid cutting into the meat.

7. Insert a clove in the intersection of the cross of each diamond on the surface (optional).

GLAZE AND BAKING

8. Place the ham in a large baking dish. Prop handle up on edge of pan + scrunched up foil so surface of the ham is level (for more even caramelisation).

9. Squeeze the juice of 1 orange (4 quarters) over the ham. Then place them along with the

remaining orange into the baking dish around the ham.

10. Brush / spoon half the glaze all over the surface and cut face of the ham (don't worry about underside, glaze drips down into pan)

11. Pour the water in the baking dish, then place in the oven.

12. Bake for 1.5 – 2 hrs, basting very generously every 30 minutes with remainig glaze + juices in pan, or until sticky and golden.

13. Use foil patches to protect bits that brown faster than others – press on lightly, caramelisation won't peel off with the foil.

14. Allow to rest for at least 20 minutes before serving. Baste, baste, baste before serving – as the glaze in the pan cools, it thickens which means it

"paints" the ham even better – but be sure to save pan juices for drizzling.

Low FODMAP Pecan Pie with Maple Cream

Prep Time: 30 minutes

Cook time: 1 hour

Serves: 10-12 people

Ingredients:

– 150g unsalted butter, softened

– 80g golden caster sugar

– 2 large egg yolks, lightly beaten

– 250g LoFo Pantry Low FODMAP plain flour, plus extra for dusting

For the filling

- 250g pecans, toasted

- 3 large eggs

- 55g golden caster sugar

- 100g golden syrup

- 50g unsalted butter, melted

- ½ tsp sea salt, plus extra for sprinkling

- 1 tbsp vanilla extract

- 1 tbsp bourbon whisky (optional)

For the maple cream

- 300ml Lactose free cream – whipped

- 3 tbsp maple syrup

Preparations

1. To make the pastry, beat the butter and sugar together in a large bowl until light and fluffy, then

beat in the egg yolks. Stir in the flour, then use your hands to bring the mixture together into a dough. Remove from the bowl, wrap and transfer to the fridge to chill for at least 1 hr.

2. Roll the pastry out onto a lightly floured surface to the thickness of a £1 coin, then lift into a 23cm loose-bottomed tart tin. Press the pastry into the base and sides of the tin, allowing any excess to hang over the sides. Put the tin on a baking sheet and chill for 30 mins.

3. Heat the oven to 180C

4. Prick the base of the pastry case with a fork. Line with baking parchment and baking beans and bake for 20 mins, then remove the parchment and beans and bake for 10-15 mins more until golden. Remove from the oven and leave to cool in the tin before using a small serrated knife to trim away the excess pastry.

5. To make the filling, roughly chop or bash half the pecans and set aside. Whisk the eggs and sugar together in a large bowl, then add the golden syrup, butter, salt, vanilla extract and bourbon, if using, and continue to whisk until everything is well combined. Add the pecans and mix again to thoroughly combine.

6. Pour the pecan filling into the pastry case and arrange the remaining whole pecans on top. Bake for 20 mins until evenly coloured – it should be lightly golden brown and set with a slight wobble when you gently shake the tin. Remove from the oven and set aside to cool for at least 1 hr. Just before serving, whip the cream and maple syrup together to soft peaks and serve alongside the pie.

Low FODMAP Moussaka

Prep Time: 30 minutes

Cook time: 1hr 45 minutes

Serves: 6-8

Ingredients

150g red capsicum, halved lengthways, seeds removed

2 Tbs olive oil, plus extra as needed

3 large eggplants, cut lengthways into 5 mm-thick slices

500 g minced pork

500 g minced lamb

1 tsp cumin seeds

1 tsp ground cinnamon

1 tbsp dried oregano

1 tsp ground cardamom

2 tsp FreeFOD Low FODMAP Onion Replacer

2 tsp FreeFOD Low FODMAP Garlic Replacer

800 g tinned crushed tomatoes

120g Liddells Lactose free parmesan

Béchamel

750 ml(3 cups) Liddells lactose free milk

4 cloves and 1 bay leaf

100 g unsalted butter

75 g (½ cup) LoFo Pantry Low FODMAP plain flour

Preparations

Resting time 10 minutes

1. Preheat the oven to 180°C (160°C fan-forced).

2. Flatten the capsicum halves with the palm of your hand, then place, skin-side up, on baking trays lined with foil and grill on the highest oven shelf for 15 minutes or until the skins are blistered black (see Note). Pull the sides of the foil to the centre over the capsicum and fold to enclose it completely. Leave to steam for 10 minutes, then peel and discard the skin and finely chop the flesh. Set aside.

3. Meanwhile, heat a drizzle of olive oil on a cast-iron grill-plate over high heat until smoking. Working in batches, grill the eggplant slices for 30 seconds on each side or until both sides have clear char marks, adding extra oil as needed; as the grill-plate heats, it will take less time to grill.

4. Heat 1 tablespoon of the olive oil in a large non-stick frying pan over high heat and cook the mince,

stirring for 6–8 minutes or until the meat is brown. Add the cumin, cinnamon, oregano and cardamom, then, stirring continuously, cook for another 5 minutes. Season to taste with salt and pepper and set aside.

5. Heat the remaining olive oil in a large heavy-based frying pan over medium heat and cook the onion and garlic replacer for 4 minutes or until soft and translucent. Add the capsicum and tomato and bring to a simmer, then cook for 15–20 minutes, stirring occasionally. Add to the mince mixture, then simmer over low heat for 15 minutes. Season to taste.

6. Meanwhile, to make the béchamel, place the milk and clove-studded onion in a small heavy-based saucepan and bring to a simmer over medium heat. Melt the butter in a non-stick saucepan over medium heat. Stir in the flour and

cook, stirring continuously, for 1 minute. Strain the milk, discarding the onion, then add 60 ml (¼ cup) of the hot milk at a time to the butter and flour mixture, whisking continuously to ensure the mixture is smooth; when all the milk is added, the sauce should be thick. If not, continue to cook for 2–3 minutes or until it has thickened. Season the sauce to taste with salt, stir and set aside.

7. To assemble, place one-third of the meat mixture in a large baking dish, top with one-third of the eggplant, then repeat the layering process until all the eggplant and meat are used. Spread the warm béchamel sauce evenly over the surface and sprinkle with the parmesan.

8. Bake the moussaka for 35 minutes or until heated through and golden brown on top. Serve immediately.

Low FODMAP Spicy Cajun Chips

Prep Time: 10 minutes

Cook time: 45 minutes

Serves: 4

Ingredients:

- 5 medium to large potatoes

- 1.5tsp PANTORI Cajun Spice blend

- 4tbsp Cooking Oil

Preparations

1. Pre-heat your oven to 200°C and line a baking tray with baking paper.

2. Peel the potatoes and cut them into chip sizes – not wedges but not as thin as fries.

3. Pop them in a large pan and cover with water and a good sprinkling of salt. Over a medium to high heat bring to a boil.

4. Leave boiling for 1 minute then drain immediately.

5. In a bowl add the oil and 1tsp of the Cajun spice blend and mix well, coat the chips and spread evenly across the baking tray.

6. Cook the chips in the oven for 40 minutes, turning them over halfway through.

7. Once removed from the oven sprinkle over the remaining half tsp of Cajun spice blend and season with salt to taste.

8. Serve with a Tangy Cajun Mayo – to make this, mix 2 TBS mayonnaise with a little of the Cajun Spice Blend and a squeeze of lime.

LOW-FODMAP RECIPES FOR DINNER

Low FODMAP Miso Sesame Glazed Eggplant Chips

Prep time: 20 mins

Cook time: 25 mins

Serves: 4

Ingredients:

• 2 eggplants

• A handful of sesame seeds

Marinade:

• ¼ cup white miso

• 1 tbsp soy sauce

• 3 tbsp garlic infused olive oil

• Salt (a pinch)

Dipping sauce:

• Sesame Roasted Kewpie Mayo

Preparations

1. Combine and mix the marinade ingredients in one bowl

2. Cut the eggplant in half and then into 4 four quarter wedges

3. Coat the eggplant with the marinade

4. Sprinkle sesame seeds over the top

5. Place in the air fryer on 180°C for 20-25 minutes, flipping the eggplants half way through

6. Serve warm with sesame roasted kewpie mayo drizzled over the top.

Low FODMAP Rice Pilaf

Prep Time: 15 minutes

Cook time: 60 minutes

Serves: 4

Ingredients:

• 3 Carrots, quartered lengthways

• 2 Courgettes, cut into similar lengths to the carrot

• 150g Green beans, ends trimmed & sliced in half lengthways

• 4 Spring onions, green ends only, finely sliced

• 1 tbsp cumin seeds, Plus a little extra.

• 3 tbsp olive oil

• 30g Almond flakes

• 50g Raisins

- 2tsp Pantori vegetable bouillon

- 525ml cold water

- 300g basmati rice

- Coconut yoghurt to serve

- Handful of Parsley, chopped

- Salt and pepper

- 80g Pomegranate seeds (optional)

- 1 lemon cut into wedges

To serve:

– 1 Cheese slice or vegan alternative (optional)

– 200g Fries to serve (optional)

Preparations

For the roasted vegetables:

1. Preheat the oven to Fan 180°C and line a large baking tray with baking paper. Spread the carrots

out on the tray, drizzle with oil and a sprinkling of cumin seeds, and season lightly with salt and pepper. Roast in the oven for 20 minutes.

2. Remove from the oven and add the courgettes to the tray, tossing carefully with the carrot. Return to the oven for a further 10 minutes.

3. Finally, add the green beans to the tray and toss once more before returning to the oven for a final 20 minutes.

4. Remove the vegetables from the oven and use to top your Rice pilaf.

For the Rice pilaf:

1. Whilst the vegetables are roasting for its final 20 minutes, you can start the rice. In a bowl soak your rice in cold water, give it a good stir and then drain.

2. In a large saucepan over medium heat, warm 2 tbsp of oil. Add the Spring onions and 1tbsp of cumin seeds and cook for 1 minute. Add the rice and continue to cook for another 2-3 minutes.

3. Add in the vegetable bouillon, the water and stir. Turn up the heat to bring to a boil. Cover with a lid, reduce the heat to LOW and cook for 10 minutes until almost tender.

4. Remove from the heat, and fluff up with a fork, stir through the raisins and place the lid back on and set aside for 5 minutes to steam.

5. Stir in half of the flaked almonds and season to taste.

6. When serving sprinkle over the chopped parsley and remainder of the almond flakes. If you also have pomegranate seeds sprinkle them over at this point.

7. Top with the roasted vegetables and a drizzle of coconut yoghurt and serve with wedges of lemon.

This recipe is low FODMAP when divided into 4 serves. Whilst you may want to go back for more and more, keep in mind that 1 serve in considered low in FODMAP and excess consumption may trigger symptom development.

Low FODMAP Soba Noodle Stir Fry

Prep time: 15 minutes

Cook time: 20-25 minutes

Serves: 2

Ingredients:

– Garlic infused olive oil

- 200g beef sliced

- 1 cup Bok Choy (roughly chopped)

- 1 cup Gai Ian / Chinese broccoli

- 2 carrots (grated)

- 1 small red capsicum

- 16g spring onion (green part only)

- Ginger (small piece, finely chopped)

- Coriander (chopped)

- 180g Soba Noodles (wheat or buckwheat)

Sauce

- 2 Tbsp. Soy sauce

- 2 Tbsp. Slightly Different Foods Sweet Chilli Sauce

- Pinch of sesame seeds

Preparations

1. Fry beef slices in garlic infused olive oil

2. Once beef turns brown, add in Bok Choy, Chinese broccoli, carrot and capsicum into fry pan, and cook on medium-high for about 10-15 minutes.

3. Add in the greens of spring onion and ginger.

4. Cook Soba noodles according to packet instructions.

5. Mix sauce ingredients together, add to stir fry and top with chopped coriander to serve.

Mediterranean Mezze

Prep time: 20 minutes

Cook time: 7-10 minutes

Serves: 4 (alongside many other dishes served at parties and gatherings)

Ingredients:

- 4 Gem lettuce leaves

- 4 Tender stem broccoli

- 4 Radishes

- 1 Pack of halloumi

- 1 Corn-on-the-cob

- 1 Bell pepper (red or green)

- ½ Large or one small courgette

- ½ Aubergine

- 30g Watercress

To Serve:

- Small pot of Bay's Kitchen Maple Chipotle Vegan Mayonnaise

– Small pot of Bay's Kitchen Garden Herb Vegan Mayonnaise

– Small pot of Bay's Kitchen Tomato Ketchup with Sundried Tomatoes

– Small pot of Bay's Kitchen BBQ Sauce with Smoked Paprika

(Low FODMAP serve for each is 20g)

Preparations

1. Firstly, prepare your vegetables – chop or slice the pepper into long strips or square pieces. Cut the aubergine length ways into long slices. Chop the corn-on-the-cob into 4 equal sections. Slice the courgette into pieces and halve again (leave whole if using a BBQ as halves will be too small!). Chop your radishes or cut into them multiple times but not all the way through to create flower type design.

2. Slice your halloumi into 8 equal slices.

3. Heat a griddle pan (or regular frying pan if you don't have a griddle, or use the BBQ!) and add a splash of oil.

4. The corn-on-the-cob takes the longest to cook so add that to the pan first. After about 2 mins, add the other vegetables. Continue to turn to griddle both sides evenly.

5. After another couple of minutes add the halloumi. Again keep turning to get an even griddle on both sides. Cook for 2-3 minutes until golden brown.

6. Once done, remove all the food from the heat.

7. Arrange the lettuce and corn-on-the-cobs first onto a serving platter, then add the halloumi cheese. Then add the rest of the veggies,

alternating between them all. Add the watercress and your done!

8. Serve with pots of Bay's Kitchen's condiments for dipping.

Griddled Vegetable Burger

Prep time: 5 minutes

Cook time: 20 minutes

Serves: 2

Ingredients:

- 30g Bay's Kitchen Maple & Chipotle Vegan Mayonnaise or Bay's Kitchen Garden Herb Mayonnaise

- 2 Gluten free burger buns

- 6 Gem lettuce Leaves

- ½ Bell pepper (red or green)

- ½ Large or one small courgette

- ½ Aubergine

- 90g Tender stem broccoli

- 4 Oyster mushrooms

- Splash of oil (olive or garlic-infused work well)

To serve:

- 1 Cheese slice or vegan alternative (optional)

- 200g Fries to serve (optional)

Preparations

1. If serving with fries, remember to factor in the cooking of these with your timings.

2. Prepare your vegetables – slice the half pepper into long strips. Cut the aubergine and courgette

length ways into long slices. Cut the mushrooms in half or remove the stalks if you prefer not to have these.

3. Heat a griddle pan (or regular frying pan if you don't have a griddle, or use the BBQ!) and add a splash of oil.

4. The broccoli takes the longest to cook so add that to the pan and then 30seconds to a minute later add the other vegetables.

5. Turn the veggies so they are charred on both sides and remove form the heat once cooked to your liking.

6. Slice the bun and toast on the griddle for about 30 seconds on each side.

7. Remove the bun from the griddle and place it on your plate, drizzle half the mayonnaise to the base of the buns.

8. Add the lettuce leaves and then layer up with your griddled vegetables.

9. Drizzle the remainder of the mayonnaise on top.

10. If using, add the cheese and then place the top of the bun on top to finish!

11. Serve with fries and why not try Bay's Kitchen Tomato Ketchup or BBQ for dipping?!

Eggplant and Zucchini Pasta

Prep time: 5 minutes

Cook time: 15 minutes

Serves: 3

Ingredients:

- ½ cup diced zucchini

- ½ cup diced carrot

- ½ cup diced eggplant

- Cheddar cheese (to garnish)

- ¾ cup gluten free pasta

- ¼ cup cherry tomatoes

- Olive oil

- ½ tsp black pepper

- ½ tsp paprika

- ½ tsp oregano

- Salt to taste

- Arugula (optional)

Method:.

Add your pasta to a pot filled with boiling water and let it boil for 7 minutes until al dente (or follow specific cooking instructions on the packet). Add a pinch of salt.

While the pasta is cooking, chop the carrot, zucchini, cherry tomatoes, and eggplant into small cubes and sauté in a pan with olive oil for 5-7 mins.

Add the black pepper, paprika and salt.

Drain the pasta and add to the sautéed vegetables. Stir well to combine.

Garnish with some grated cheddar cheese, oregano and some fresh basil leaves if you like.

Serve the pasta with some arugula on the side and enjoy!

Prawn Curry

Prep time: 5 minutes

Cook time: 25 minutes

Serves: 4

<u>Ingredients:</u>

- 60g (8-10) large, uncooked, peeled prawns

- 10g peanuts

- ½ small red Capsicum

- 3 medium cherry tomatoes

- 2 tbsp shredded coconut

- ¼ tsp garam masala

- ½ tsp turmeric powder

- ½ tsp coriander powder

- ½ tsp cumin powder

- 3 tbsp water

- 2 ½ tbsp olive oil

- Coriander leaves (optional garnish)

- 1 cup cooked brown or basmati rice

Preparations

1. In a blender, add the red capsicum, cherry tomatoes, peanuts, shredded coconut, and 3 tbsp of water and blend together until smooth.

2. In a heated pan, add 2 ½ tbsp of olive oil and the blended mix. Keep stirring for about 5 minutes, ensuring it does not form lumps or stick to the pan.

3. Add the garam masala, turmeric powder, coriander powder, cumin powder and salt to the pan and mix well.

4. Now add the prawns into the pan and cook for 5-8 minutes on low heat. Add 1-2 tbsp of water if the sauce starts to thicken too much.

5. Turn off the heat and garnish with coriander leaves (optional) and serve with rice! Enjoy!

Vegetarian Chilli Corn Carne

Prep time: 15 minutes

Cook time: 1.5 hours

Serves: 4-5 people

<u>Ingredients:</u>

• 3 large Red Peppers/Capsicum – roughly chopped, (4cm)

• 4 Spring Onions – green ends only

• Olive oil

• 200g tinned Chickpeas – rinsed & drained

- 1 Jar low FODMAP Passata

- Handful of fresh Coriander (10g) – finely chopped

- 1 Aubergine/Eggplant – cut into chunks, (4cm)

- 1 large Carrot – grated

- 1 stalk Celery – finely diced

- Mug of Coffee (decaf if preferred)

- 20g Pantori Chilli con Carne spice blend

Preparations

1. Pre-heat the oven to 200C, line a baking try with baking paper.

2. Toss the Aubergine and red pepper in oil and 1tsp of your Pantori chilli blend and spread evenly across the tray, roast in the oven for 20 minutes.

3. In the meantime, heat 1 tbsp of oil in a large saucepan over a medium heat.

4. Add the carrot, celery, spring onions and sweat on a medium heat for 10 minutes, stirring regularly.

5. Add the aubergine and peppers to the pan and combine.

6. Add the remaining spice blend and stir to coat the mixture.

7. Pour in the coffee and passata, stir and turn the heat to low and simmer for 30-40 minutes uncovered, stirring occasionally.

8. Drain and rinse the chickpeas, add into the chilli and simmer for 10 minutes.

9. Service with rice and a teaspoon of sour cream or your favourite accompaniments.Winter nights call for chilli con carne, and what's better than one packed full of vegetables and flavour?

Asian Noodle Broth

Prep time: 15 minutes

Cook time: 10 minutes

Serves: 5-6

<u>Ingredients:</u>

Pantori Mushroom bouillon – 4 tsp in 2.5 litres of boiling wate

Thumb sized piece of ginger – peeled and chopped finely

1 Star Anise

6 Radishes – finely sliced

2 Bok/Pak Choi – Weighing less than 300g in total, each leaf sliced in half lengthways

1 large Carrot – Peeled into strips

3tbsp Gluten Free Soy sauce / tamari

2tbsp Fish sauce

4 Spring onions – green ends only – finely sliced

Large handful of bean sprouts

1-2 Chillies – sliced (your preference on heat levels)

Coriander – leaves removed for garnish and stalks finely chopped

About 300g of rice noodles – I prefer the wide over vermicelli

<u>Preparations</u>

1. In a large saucepan on a medium-high heat bring your two litres of mushroom stock to a boil.

2. Add the star anise, ginger, soy sauce and fish sauce to the stock and keep on a very gentle

simmer on a low heat while you prep the other ingredients.

3. To prep the carrot, use a peeler and rotating the carrot peel off fine strips of carrot and put to the side with the rest of your prepped veg.

4. With the stock simmering add in your noodles to begin to soften.

5. After 1 minute add in the radish, carrot, bok choi, bean sprouts and chopped coriander stalks.

6. Give it a couple of minutes simmering until the noodles have cooked through.

7. Serve and garnish with sliced chilli (to your liking), spring onions and coriander.

8. Enjoy!

Low FODMAP Homemade Veggie Pizza

Prep time: 15 minutes

Cook time: 10 minutes

Serves: 2

Ingredients:

– ½ Jar Bay's Kitchen Tomato & Basil Sauce

– 1 Gluten free, low FODMAP pizza base (shop-bought or homemade)

– 4 Tender stem broccoli

– 85g Sliced red pepper

– 1 Asparagus spear

– 1 Small sliced courgette

– 30g Mozzarella (or plant-based alternative)

– Fresh Basil for garnish

<u>**Preparations**</u>

1. 1. If using a homemade pizza base, remember to factor this into the preparation and cook times.

2. Prepare your vegetables – slice the half pepper into long strips. Cut the courgette lengthways into long slices. Heat a griddle pan (or regular frying pan if you don't have a griddle, or use the BBQ!) and add a splash of oil.

3. Lightly griddle the vegetables until al dente.

4. Spread the Bay's Kitchen Tomato & Basil Stir-in Sauce onto the gluten free pizza base, making sure that it is even.

5. Sprinkle with cheese and arrange the cooked vegetables onto the pizza.

6. Cook the pizza at 180 degrees for 8-10 minutes (depending on pizza base instructions/recipe you're using).

7. Add fresh basil leaves and serve.

This recipe is classified as low FODMAP when divided into 2 servings. Like any meal, it is recommended you know your FODMAP friendly portion sizes.

Garden Vegetable Pasta

Prep time: 10 minutes

Cook time: 20 minutes

Serves: 4

<u>Ingredients:</u>

– 1 package Orgran Garden Veggie Penne 300g

– 500g low FODMAP tomato passata sauce (without onion or garlic)

- 1 green zucchini, sliced

- 1 eggplant, roughly chopped

- 4 squash, sliced

- 1 tbsp olive oil

- Salt and Pepper to taste

- Fresh basil and parmesan, to serve

Preparations

1. Bring a pot of salted water to the boil and cook pasta per instructions. Drain and set aside.

2. In a large saucepan, fry zucchini, eggplant, and squash with the olive oil, until soft and cooked through. Add the passata sauce and stir until a light simmer. Add the salt and pepper and mix for 2-3 minutes.

3. Stir through the cooked pasta and top with fresh basil and parmesan to serve.

Cajan Chicken Skewers

Prep time: 15 minutes

Cook time: 10 minutes

Serves: 4-5

Ingredients:

4 or 5 Chicken breasts (1 per person)

2 tbsp Oil

20g Pantori Cajun Spice Blend

Preparations

1. Soak your skewers in water and set aside.

2. Cut your chicken into 2cm cubes.

3. In a bowl toss the chicken in the oil & spice blend and leave to marinate for at least 10 minutes.

4. Thread the chicken pieces onto your skewers.

5. Heat a griddle pan over a medium heat and cook the skewers for 8-10 minutes, or until cooked through, turning frequently.

Crispy Cornflake Chicken

Prep time: 5 minutes

Cook time: 20-25 minutes

Serves: 2

Ingredients:

2 chicken breast – cut into 5 strips

2 heaped tbsp Coconut yoghurt (approx. 60g)

10g PANTORI Fajita Spice blend

75g Cornflakes – Crush to a crumb but not quite a powder

<u>Preparations</u>

1. Pre-heat your oven to 200°C/ 392°F, line a baking tray with foil or baking paper to sit underneath a wire rack.

2. In a bowl mix together the coconut yoghurt and 1tsp of the fajita spice blend, add in the chicken strips and coat well.

3. Tip your crushed cornflakes onto a plate and mix the remainder of the spice blend in and coat the chicken evenly, pop them on the wire rack in the oven and bake for 18 minutes until they are nice and crispy, and the chicken is cooked through.

4. For a dip we like to add a sprinkling of the Fajita spice blend into mayonnaise and a squeeze of lime for a spicy, tangy dip.

Low FODMAP Hunter's Chicken

Prep time: 5 minutes

Cook time: 25 minutes

Serves: 2

<u>Ingredients:</u>

40g Bay's Kitchen BBQ Sauce with Smoked Paprika

2 Chicken Breasts

4 Rashers smoked back bacon

25g Grated Cheddar Cheese

25g Grated Mozzarella

Olive Oil

Sea salt and freshly ground black pepper

<u>Preparations</u>

1. Oil a roasting dish and add in the chicken breasts and bacon. Season with salt and pepper. Cook at 200C/180C fan for 20 minutes, or until the chicken is cooked through.

2. Once the chicken is cooked, pour the Bay's Kitchen BBQ Sauce over the top and sprinkle over the cheese.

3. Place back in the oven for 5 minutes until the cheese is melted and the sauce is bubbling.

4. Serve with your favourite Low FODMAP sides.

Low FODMAP Green Curry

Prep time: 10 mins

Cook time: 20 mins

Serves: 2

Ingredients:

350 g of chicken or meat of your choice or firm tofu

200g FODMAPPED For You Green Curry Simmer Sauce

Half a carrot

Quarter of a red capsicum

Six green beans

Half cup of broccoli

1 tablespoon of olive oil

Three-quarter cup of basmati rice

One lime

Coriander

<u>Preparations</u>

1. In a pan add 1 tablespoon of oil

2. Once the oil is hot add the chicken or meat of choice and cook for 3 to 4 minutes or until the meat is almost cooked then remove the meat from the pan

3. Add the carrot into the pan and cook for 2 to 3 minutes

4. Then add the rest of the veggies and sauté for 2 to 3 minutes.

5. Cover the veggies with with a lid to steam for another 3-5 minutes or until they're cooked

6. Once the vegetables are cooked add the meat back into the pan and pour 200 g of the

FODMAPPED Green Curry Simmer Sauce and stir through

7. Let this simmer and cook for a further 12 to 15 minutes

8. Serve with steamed basmati rice and garnish with a lime wedge and chopped coriander.

9. Enjoy!

LOW-FODMAP RECIPES FOR SALAD

Low FODMAP Chicken & Bacon Caesar Salad

Prep time: 5 minutes

Cook time: 20 minutes

Serves: 2

Ingredients:

- 2 Tbsp Bay's Kitchen Garden Herb Vegan Mayonnaise

- 2 Chicken breast or vegan alternative

- 30g Parmesan shavings or vegan alternative

- 20g Bacon lardons or vegan alternative

- 20g Gluten free croutons

- 8 Romaine lettuce leaves

– 5ml Olive oil

– Seasoning for chicken (optional)

<u>Preparations</u>

1. Preheat the oven to 200°C, 180°C fan.

2. Using a meat mallet or rolling pin, pound each chicken breast to pprox.. 2cm at the thickest part (this just helps even cooking).

3. Line a baking pan with foil or baking parchment and place the chicken in. You can season with salt and pepper, or even your favourite herbs, like rosemary or oregano.

4. Once the oven is up to temperature, bake the chicken for 18-20 mins.

5. Whilst the chicken is cooking you can prepare the rest of the salad. Shred the lettuce and share evenly between two bowls.

6. Drizzle half of the mayonnaise evenly across the two bowls.

7. Preheat 5ml of oil in a frying pan on a medium to high heat, then add the bacon lardons. Continue to turn the lardons regularly to ensure they get equally crispy. Fry for pprox.. 5 mins.

8. Once your chicken is cooked, remove from the over and then slice into 1cm wide strips or roughly chop – whichever you prefer!

9. Add the chicken and the lardons on top of the lettuce and then drizzle the remainder of the mayonnaise on top.

10. Finish with the croutons and parmesan!

Low FODMAP Beetroot and Roast Pumpkin Salad

Prep time: 20 mins

Cook time: 30 mins

Serves: 4

<u>Ingredients:</u>

- 500g Pumpkin

- 2 large Beetroots

- 2 tbsp. Olive oil

- Salt and Pepper

- 100g Rocket

- 150g Snap Peas

- 100g Feta

- 1 cup Pine Nuts

- 2 Mandarin

Citrus Maple Dijon Dressing:

Ingredients:

3 tablespoons olive oil

2 tablespoons pure maple syrup

1 tablespoon Dijon mustard

2 tablespoons freshly squeezed orange juice

1 tablespoon lemon juice

Salt and pepper to taste

Preparations

1. In a small bowl, whisk together the olive oil, maple syrup, Dijon mustard, orange juice, and lemon juice until well combined.

2. Season with salt and pepper to taste.

3. Taste the dressing and adjust the sweetness or acidity according to your preference. You can add a bit more maple syrup for sweetness or lemon juice for acidity.

Preparations

1: Preheat oven to 200°C.

2: Chop pumpkin into cubes, then peel and chop beetroot into cubes.

3: Place prepared pumpkin and beetroot onto lined baking trays. Drizzle with oil to coat and season with salt and pepper to taste. Bake for 30 minutes or until vegetables are tender and slightly browned. Remove from tray and set aside to cool slightly.

4: Leave oven on and toast pine nuts for 5-10 minutes or until browned

5: Peel and divide mandarins

6: Meanwhile, place all of the dressing ingredients into a small bowl and whisk to combine.

7: To assemble, place the rocket on a serving platter and top with the roasted vegetables, mandarin, pine nuts and sugar snap peas.

8: Finish with crumbled Feta and a drizzle of the dressing and enjoy!

Low FODMAP Roasted Sweet potato and Lemon Chicken Salad

Prep Time: 30 mins

Rest time: 1 hour

Cook time: 40 mins

Serves: 2

<u>**Ingredients:**</u>

100g Boneless chicken breast

1 tsp Garlic-infused olive oil

1 tbsp Lemon, juiced

1 tsp Lemon rind

½ tsp Oregano, ground

½ tsp Rosemary, dried

1 Sweet potato

1 tbsp Extra-virgin olive oil

Salt and Pepper

1 cup Iceberg lettuce, diced

¼ Tomato, diced

¼ Carrot, grated

¼ Cucumber, diced

1 tbsp Pomegranate seeds

Salad Dressing

1 tsp Fresh ginger, grated

1 tsp Maple Syrup

1 tbsp Lemon, juices

1 tsp Dijon mustard

1 tbsp Extra-virgin olive oil

Preparations

1. Combine garlic-infused olive oil, lemon juice, lemon, rind, oregano, and rosemary in bowl. Massage chicken in marinate and cover in fridge for at least 1 hour.

2. Preheat oven to 180°C.

3. Dice sweet potato into evenly sized cubes, coat with olive oil and season with salt and pepper. Place on a baking tray, ensuring no pieces cover

each other. Place in the oven for 40 minutes or until golden and crispy on the edges.

4. Remove marinated chicken from the fridge and fry on a pan.

5. Prepare vegetables and place lettuce, tomato, carrot, and cucumber into a salad bowl.

6. Prepare salad dressing by placing ginger, maple syrup, lemon juice, mustard, and olive oil into a jar. Seal with a lid and shake to combine.

7. Place cooked chicken on top of salad, then sprinkle roasted sweet potato, pomegranate seeds and salad dressing over the top.

8. Serve.

Low FODMAP Greek Salad Wrap

Prep time: 15 minutes

Serves: 2

Ingredients:

- 2 gluten-free wraps or large lettuce leaves

- 1/2 cucumber, diced

- 1/2 cup cherry tomatoes, halved

- 15 olives, pitted and sliced

- 40g crumbled feta cheese (omit for a dairy-free or vegan option)

- 2 tablespoons extra-virgin olive oil

- 1 tablespoon red wine vinegar

- 1 teaspoon dried oregano

- Salt and pepper, to taste

– Beef, Chicken or Lamb (omit for a dairy-free or vegan option)

<u>Preparations</u>

1. In a medium bowl, combine the cucumber, cherry tomatoes, olives, feta cheese (if desired), extra-virgin olive oil, red wine vinegar, dried oregano, salt, and pepper. Toss well to combine.2. Lay out the gluten-free wraps or lettuce leaves on a clean surface.3. Spoon the Greek salad mixture onto the centre of each wrap or lettuce leaf, top with your meat of choice (if desired).

4. Fold in the sides of the wrap or lettuce leaf, then roll it up tightly, similar to a burrito, ensuring the filling is secure.

5. Slice the wrap in half if desired, and serve immediately.

6. Enjoy the vibrant flavours and crisp textures of the Greek Salad Wrap. It's a refreshing and

satisfying option that brings together the classic elements of a Greek salad in a convenient handheld form.

Low FODMAP Grilled Chicken and Quinoa Salad with Lemon-Tahini Dressing

Prep time: 15 mins

Cook time: 20 minutes

Serves: 4

<u>Ingredients:</u>

For the Salad:

– 2 boneless, skinless chicken breasts

– 1 cup quinoa, rinsed

- 1 cucumber, diced

- 1 cup cherry tomatoes, halved

- 1 red bell pepper, diced

- 2 cups mixed salad greens (e.g., spinach, arugula)

- 1/4 cup chopped fresh parsley (optional for garnish)

For the Lemon-Tahini Dressing:

- 2 tablespoons tahini

- 2 tablespoons extra-virgin olive oil

- 2 tablespoons fresh lemon juice

- 1 tablespoon maple syrup

- 1 teaspoon Dijon mustard

- Salt and pepper to taste

<u>Preparations</u>

1. Prepare the Quinoa:

- In a medium saucepan, combine quinoa with 2 cups of water. Bring to a boil, then reduce heat to low, cover, and simmer for 15 minutes or until the quinoa is cooked and water is absorbed. Fluff with a fork and set aside.

2. Grill the Chicken:

- Season chicken breasts with salt and pepper. Grill over medium heat for about 6-8 minutes per side or until fully cooked. Let them rest for a few minutes, then slice into strips.

3. Prepare the Vegetables:

- In a large bowl, combine the cooked quinoa, diced cucumber, cherry tomatoes, diced red bell pepper, and mixed salad greens.

4. Make the Dressing:

- In a small bowl, whisk together tahini, olive oil, lemon juice, maple syrup, Dijon mustard, salt, and pepper until smooth.

5. Assemble the Salad:

- Add the sliced grilled chicken to the bowl with vegetables and quinoa.

- Drizzle the lemon-tahini dressing over the salad and toss gently to combine.

6. Serve:

Low FODMAP Caprese Salad Skewers

Prep time: 15 mins

Assemble time: 15 mins

Serves: 2

<u>**Ingredients:**</u>

– 12 Cherry tomatoes

– 6 Fresh mozzarella balls

– 12 Basil leaves

– 1 TBS Balsamic glaze

– 6 Toothpicks for skewering

<u>**Preparations**</u>

1. Wash and dry cherry tomatoes and basil leaves.

2. Assemble each skewer by threading a cherry tomato, a mozzarella ball, and a basil leaf onto a toothpick.

3. Repeat until you have the desired number of skewers.

4. Arrange the skewers on a serving plate or platter.

5. Drizzle with balsamic glaze just before serving.

6. Enjoy your Low FODMAP Caprese Salad Skewers!

Lo w FODMAP Sweet and Salty Grilled Bok Choy + Cucumber Salad

Serves 4

<u>Ingredients:</u>

Dressing

¼ cup (50mL) Niulife Organic Naked Coconut Amino Sauce

¼ cup (55g) tahini

2 tablespoons of toasted sesame oil

¼ cup apple cider vinegar

¼ cup avocado oil or olive oil

Salad

1 tsp coconut oil

6 heads bok choy, sliced and washed

1 tablespoon of Niulife Organic Naked Coconut Amino Sauce

2 cucumbers, chopped

2 carrots, spiralised

1 tablespoon sesame seeds, black or white

½ cup coriander, chopped

3 spring onions, green parts only, finely sliced

<u>Preparations</u>

1. Prepare the dressing by combining all the ingredients in a small bowl or jar and whisking continuously until you get a smooth homogeneous

mixture. It may seem like it's not coming together but it will.

2. Place the cucumbers, carrot, sesame seeds, coriander and spring onion in a large bowl. Pour in half the dressing and toss to coat. Set aside.

3. Heat a skillet over a high heat and add the coconut oil. Add in the bok choy and stir fry for about 30 seconds. Pour over the coconut aminos and continue to stir fry for another 30-60 seconds. Serve the bok choy on a large platter.

4. Spoon over the tossed salad mixture and drizzle over some extra dressing. Top with extra sesame seeds to serve.

www.ingramcontent.com/pod-product-compliance
Lightning Source LLC
Chambersburg PA
CBHW061043250726

48653CB00001B/230